Body Scrubs for Gorgeous Skin: DIY All Natural Beauty Secrets For Skin Like Jennifer Aniston's

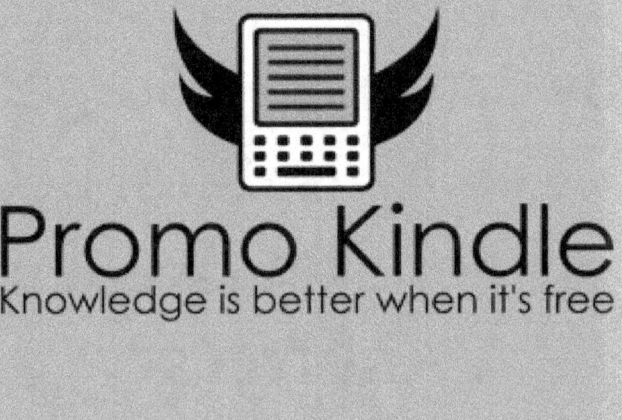

Disclaimer and Terms of Use: Effort has been made to ensure that the information in this book is accurate and complete, however, the author and the publisher do not warrant the accuracy of the information, text and graphics contained within the book due to the rapidly changing nature of science, research, known and unknown facts and internet. The Author and the publisher do not hold any responsibility for errors, omissions or contrary interpretation of the subject matter herein. This book is presented solely for motivational and informational purposes only.

Table of Contents

Fingers and Toes

Tallow Blend Balm

Ingredients:
- ¼ C grass fed beef lard
- 2 ½ tsp olive oil
- 3 drops lavender oil

Directions: You want to use a glass container and microwave down the lard, masons jars work great. Stir the olive oil and lavender in next, and move to refrigerator and let this set. You want a balm like substance. Once this hardens take it out of the fridge and store with light tightly.

Hand Sanitizer

Ingredients:
- 2 T aloe Vera
- 1 T water
- 1/8 tsp Vitamin E
- 5 drops thieves oil

Directions: Take a small squeeze bottle and use this to store the sanitizer. Add everything together in a little water. You don't want this really thick, so you can add more water if you need but not too much.

Ingredients:
- Spray bottle
- Water
- 2 T aloe Vera
- Few drops of vitamin E
- 30 drops of lemon, lime, lavender, melaleuca

Directions: Fill the bottle with water, at least half way. Add the vitamin, aloe and oils, and shake well.

Foam hand wash

Ingredients:
- 1/3 C liquid no scent castile soap
- 2/3 C water
- 1/8 tsp essential peppermint oil

Directions: Add the soap to a jar or bottle, add the oil to the jar and stir and combine. Fill the rest of the jar or bottle with water, add lid and pumper and you are good to go.

Peppermint Foot Soak

Ingredients:
- 1 ½ C sea salt
- 14 drops peppermint essential oil
- 1 dap vitamin E oil

Directions: Add everything together and you only have to use about 1-2 T per foot bath.

All natural hand soap

Ingredients:
- 12 oz. almond milk
- 3 oz. lye
- 10 oz. coconut milk
- 12 oz. lard
- ½ oz. essential oil

Directions: In a small or medium size bowl add the partially frozen milk and lye with spoon. On low to medium heat melt the coconut oil, lard and oil. Slowly add the melted mix and lye and blend for 10 minutes then let sit for 10 minutes. Pour into molds and let dry for 24 hours.

Sea salt hand or feet scrub

Ingredients:
- 1 C fine sea salt
- ½ C oil
- 10 drops essential oils

Directions: Mix everything together in a canning jar, or small bowl and store in air tight, screw top container. Apply to hands or feet and add make sure to rinse with warm water.

Pump Hand soap

Ingredients:

- Castile soap
- Distilled water
- Foaming dispenser

Directions: Fill dispenser, with a little of the soap, about 1 T. fill the rest of the bottle with water.

Face creams and washes

Perfect skin Cream

Ingredients:
- 2 Tgrapeseed oil
- 1 T borage seed oil
- T hazelnut oil
- 1 T hemp seed oil
- 20 drops frankincense

Directions: Mix everything together in a dark jar or glass and store in cool dark place, sealed.

Ingredients:
- 2 T coconut oil
- 4 drop purification oil blend

Directions: in small saucepan melt coconut oil and remove from heat then add purification oil. Stir slowly, and you can use eye dropped or funnel to transfer to lip balm tubes. This way you can just roll it on. But you need to let this set in cold area.

Cucumber Mask

Ingredients:
- 1 or 2 cucumbers
- 2 T unrefined coconut oil
- ¼ C aloe Vera
- 8 drops carrot seed essential oil

Directions: Mix everything until it's creamy. Spoon this into ice cube tray slots and freeze. You want to add this around the eyes for about 12 minutes or so. Don get this in your eyes though, it will burn.

Eucycalptus Shaving cream

Ingredients:
- 1/3 C coconut oil
- ½ C shea butter
- 1 T apricot oil
- 15 drops lavender
- 5 drops peppermint
- 5 drops eucalyptus
- 1 tsp baking soda

Directions: Using a glass bowl, set this on top of a saucepan of water, add coconut oil, butter and jojoba oil in the glass bowl bring the water to a boil, and whisk ingredients in glass bowl until it goes from white to clear. Remove the oils from heat and add essentials and baking soda. White and refrigerate. You can use a mixer to make light and fluffy. Set back in the fridge for about another hour. Whip again, until it looks like whipped cream. Spoon cream into jars.

Ingredients:
- 1 tsp vitamin C powder
- 1 tsp water
- 1 tsp glycerin
- 1/8 tsp vitamin E

Directions: Mix everything in a small bowl, until everything dissolves. Move to a dark glass bottle or jar with an eye dropper similar tool.

Seaweed Mask

Ingredients:
- 1 tsp honey
- 1 tsp bladder wrack powder
- ¼ tsp water

Directions: Combine seaweed and honey and add water to thin the consistency, of which you want. Start with about ¼ tsp.

Clay mask

Ingredients:
- Bentonite clay
- Unfiltered apple cider vinegar

Directions: Mix both of equal amounts and stir.

Honey face acne mask

Ingredients:
- 3 tsp raw honey
- ½ tsp cinnamon

Directions: Mix together and apply to face and trouble areas

Honey mask for dry skin

Ingredients:
- 1 tsp mashed avocado
- 1 tsp whole milk yogurt
- 1 tsp raw honey

Directions: Mix together and apply to face

Honey mask for sensitive mask

Ingredients:
- 2 tsp raw honey
- 1 tsp aloe Vera gel

Directions: Stir the aloe with the honey and apply all over, let sit and wash away.

Dark spot and scar honey mask

Ingredients:
- 2 its raw honey
- ½ tsp lemon juice

Directions: combine the lemon juice and honey and apply mixture all over your face. Let sit and let lemon juice do its work.

Makeup & mascara remover

Ingredients:
- Jojoba oil
- Castor oil
- Coconut oil

Directions: mix and scrub on face and rinse

All natural eye shadow

Ingredients:
- Arrowroot powder
- Shea butter
- Cocoa powder
- Nutmeg
- Dried beet root
- Turmeric
- Allspice

Directions: start by putting ½ tsp water in a small bowl. The more root you use the lighter the shade you can use more or less.

Ingredients:

- 2 tsp coconut oil
- 4 tsp. aloe Vera gel
- 1 capsule activated charcoal
- Or cocoa powder

Directions: ix everything together, and store in air tight container. Always use a clear brush.

All natural foundation

Ingredients:
- Arrowroot powder
- Cocoa powder
- Nutmeg
- Ground cinnamon

Directions: start with the base of root, the more root the lighter the tones. You can add any of the powders for the complexion you're needing or wanting.

All natural blush

Ingredients:
- Arrowroot hibiscus powder
- Cinnamon

Directions: add the two together, you can add different powders or less for different tones

Earthly Bronzer

Ingredients:
- 1 T ground cinnamon
- 1 tsp cocoa powder
- 1 tsp nutmeg
- 2 tsp arrow root
- 15 drops rosemary essential oils

Directions: You can adjust what you want by the color bronzer you're wanting. Mix the powders and pack firmly.

www.ingramcontent.com/pod-product-compliance
Lightning Source LLC
Chambersburg PA
CBHW070525290526
45790CB00003B/1297